COPD

THINGS YOU SHOULD KNOW
(QUESTIONS AND ANSWERS)

By Rumi Michael Leigh

Introduction

I would like to thank and congratulate you for purchasing this book, " *COPD, things you should know (questions and answers*)" series.

This book will help you understand, revise and have a good general knowledge and keywords of COPD and how it affects the lives of people who suffer from COPD.

Thanks again for purchasing this book, I hope you enjoy it !

Chapter 1

1)   What is COPD?

-    COPD is an irreversible bronchial obstruction that is characterized by chronic bronchitis and emphysema.

2)   What constitutes COPD?

-    Chronic bronchitis and emphysema.

3)   What is chronic bronchitis?

-    Chronic bronchitis is a chronic inflammation of the bronchi.

4)   What is emphysema?

-    Emphysema is the destruction of the wall of the cells by enlargement or distension.

5)   What is the difference between COPD of bronchial origin and COPD of emphysema origin?

-    In COPD of bronchial origin there is cough but in COPD of emphysema origin there is no cough.

6)   Is emphysema reversible?

-    No, emphysema is not reversible, it is irreversible.

7)   How many stages of COPD are there?

-    There are 4 stages of COPD.

8)   What are the 4 stages of COPD?

-    The 4 stages of COPD are the mild, moderate, severe and very severe stage.

9)   What is an evolutionary disease?

-    An evolutionary disease is a chronic disease that evolves over time.

10) When can we say that someone has chronic bronchitis?

- We can say that someone has chronic bronchitis when the cough lasts at least 3 months in the year and 2 years in a row without other respiratory diseases being present.

Chapter 2

1) Is COPD reversible?

\-   No, COPD is not reversible.

2) Is COPD treatable?

\-   Yes, COPD is treatable.

3) Can people with COPD have a normal life?

\-   Yes, people with COPD can have a normal life if they improve their lifestyle and follow the advice of their doctor.

4) At what age are people with COPD often diagnosed?

\-   People with COPD are often diagnosed as early as 40 years old.

5) What are the main clinical signs of COPD?

-      The main clinical signs of COPD are dyspnea, chronic cough and sputum.

6)   What always worsens the symptoms of COPD?

-      Effort always worsens the symptoms of COPD.

7)   Name a major symptom of COPD.

-      A major symptom of COPD is muscular fatigue.

8)   What are the two main clinical forms of COPD?

-      The two main clinical forms of COPD are stable COPD and acute exacerbation.

9)   What is an exacerbation?

-      An exacerbation is a worsening of the existing symptoms of a disease.

10)   What are the treatments for COPD exacerbation?

- The treatments for COPD exacerbation include treatment by bronchodilators, administration of antibiotics and systemic corticosteroids.

Chapter 3

1)   What is the tissue of the lungs?

-    The tissue of the lungs is the lung parenchyma.

2)   Name a difference between the structure of the trachea and that of bronchioles.

-    Bronchioles do not have cartilage.

3)   How many types of proteins are there in the lungs?

-    The lungs have 2 types of protein.

4)   What are the proteins of the lungs?

-    The proteins of the lungs are elastin and collagen.

5)   What are the functions of elastin in the lungs?

-      The functions of elastin are the distension and retraction of the lungs.

6)   What is the function of collagen in the lungs?

-      The function of collagen is the maintenance of the lungs.

7)   What happens when there is little elastin in the lungs?

-      When there is little elastin in the lungs, the lungs become rigid.

8)   What is the function of goblet cells?

-      Goblet cells produce mucus to trap and finally expectorate waste, it has a function of protection.

9)   What is active expirium?

-      Active expirium is the use of force to exhale.

10)   Is expirium an active process?

-	No, expirium is not an active process, it is a passive process.

Chapter 4

1) What is the pathophysiological mechanism of COPD?

- Inflammation of the bronchial tree.
- Remodeling.
- Centrilobular emphysema.

2) What does the inflammation of the bronchial tree of COPD cause?

- The inflammation of the bronchial tree of COPD causes greasy cough and whitish sputum in the morning.

3) What does remodeling of COPD cause?

- Remodeling of COPD is a decrease in bronchial lumen which causes resistance to airflow which causes dyspnea of effort.

4) What is sibilance?

- Sibilance is a noise, hissing during breathing.

5) Can we hear sibilance without a stethoscope?

- Yes, we can hear sibilance without a stethoscope.

6) What is lactic acid?

- Lactic acid is a metabolic waste produced when the muscles produce intense and prolonged efforts for a certain time.

7) What is oxidative stress?

- Oxidative stress occurs when the antioxidant systems can no longer handle the accumulation of free radicals.

8) What are free radicals?

- Free radicals are wastes produced when a part of oxygen is metabolized by our body.

9)   Does hemoglobin associate more easily with O2 or with CO2?

-      Hemoglobin easily associates with CO2.

10)   What are the complications of COPD?

-      The complications of COPD are pulmonary hypertension, lung cancer, heart disease, etc.

Chapter 5

1) What is the main cause of COPD?

- Smoking is the main cause of COPD.

2) Name 3 tobacco substances.

- Nicotine, carbon monoxide, and tars.

3) Does nicotine stimulate the sympathetic or parasympathetic system?

- Nicotine stimulates the sympathetic system.

4) Could smoking be bad for skeletal muscles?

- Yes, smoking could be bad for skeletal muscles.

5) Can passive smoking cause COPD?

- Yes, passive smoking can cause COPD.

6)   What are the effects of nicotine on the body?

-      The effect of nicotine on the body is that it increases blood pressure, leads to addiction, and damages the arteries.

7)   What is the effect of carbon monoxide on the body?

-      The effect of carbon monoxide on the body is that it causes hypoxia.

8)   How can carbon monoxide cause hypoxia?

-      Carbon monoxide causes hypoxia when it binds to hemoglobin, carboxyhemoglobin, which then decreases oxygen transport in the body.

9)   What is the effect of tars on the body?

-      The effect of tars on the body is that tars immobilize the cilia and cover the respiratory tract which reduces the gaseous exchange between the alveoli and the blood.

10)   What is the only test that provides a diagnosis of COPD?

-       The only test that provides a diagnosis of COPD is the functional respiratory test.

Chapter 6

1) What is conditioning?

- Conditioning is when a person does make enough physical effort.

2) What is reconditioning?

- Reconditioning is muscle training.

3) What kind of exercises could be suggested to a COPD patient?

- The kind of exercises that could be suggested to a COPD patient are for example, walking and cycling.

4) What is more important during reconditioning in a COPD patient?

- The intensity of the exercise is more important during reconditioning in a COPD patient.

5)   What are the origins of muscular dysfunction in COPD?

-    The origins of muscular dysfunction in COPD are smoking, physical inactivity, undernutrition, systemic inflammation, oxidative stress, etc.

6)   What are the benefits of administering oxygen to a patient in a case of COPD during exercise?

-    The benefits of administering oxygen to a patient in a case of COPD during exercise are increased endurance, decreased lactic acid, etc.

7)   What is transcutaneous electrical stimulation?

-    Transcutaneous electrical stimulation is an electrical stimulation to oxidize and increase muscle strength.

8)   Electrical stimulation is often indicated for which type of patients?

-    Electrical stimulation is often indicated for bedridden patients who do not have the means (strength) to do a physical training program and for people in critical condition.

9)   What is bronchial drainage?

-   Bronchial drainage is a technique used to remove excess mucus in the bronchi.

10)   What is FEV1?

-   Forced Expiratory Volume in 1 second.

Chapter 7

1) What is required for there to be gas exchange between the alveoli and the capillaries?

- For there to be gas exchange between the alveoli and the capillaries the ratio between perfusion and ventilation must be balanced.

2) What is perfusion?

- Perfusion is the amount of blood that reaches the capillaries of the pulmonary alveoli.

3) What is ventilation?

- Ventilation is the amount of air that reaches the pulmonary alveoli.

4) What are the respiratory volumes?

- Inspiratory reserve volume (IRV)
- Tidal volume (TV)

- Expiratory reserve volume (ERV)
- Residual volume (RV)

5) What is the value of the inspiratory reserve volume (IRV)?

- The value of the inspiratory reserve volume is 3100 ml.

6) What is the value of the tidal volume (TV)?

- The value of the tidal volume is 500 ml.

7) What is the value of the expiratory reserve volume (ERV)?

- The value of the expiratory reserve volume is 1200 ml.

8) What is the residual volume?

- Residual volume is the volume remaining in the lungs even after expiration.

9) What is the role of the residual volume?

- The role of the residual volume is to keep the alveoli open so as to avoid the collapse of the alveoli.

10) Is the residual volume in a COPD patient decreased or increased?

- The residual volume in a COPD patient is increased.

Chapter 8

1) Why is the residual volume in a COPD patient increased?

-   The residual volume in a COPD patient is increased because due to the narrowing of the airways, the air cannot be easily evacuated.

2) What is the value of the dead space in the tidal volume?

-   The value of the dead space in the tidal volume is 150 ml.

3) Name the lung capacities.

-   Inspiratory capacity (IC)
-   Functional residual capacity (FRC)
-   Vital capacity (VC)
-   Total lung capacity (TLC)

4)   What is the value of the inspiratory capacity (IC)?

-    The value of the inspiratory capacity is 3600 ml.

5)   What is the value of the functional residual capacity?

-    The value of the functional residual capacity is 2400 ml.

6)   What is the value of the vital capacity?

-    The value of the vital capacity is 4800 ml.

7)   What is the value of the total lung capacity?

-    The value of the total lung capacity is 6000 ml.

8)   What are the respiratory volumes in the inspiratory capacity?

-    The inspiratory reserve volume (3100 ml) and the tidal volume (500 ml).

9)   What are the respiratory volumes in the functional residual capacity?

-    The expiratory reserve volume (1200 ml) and the residual volume (1200 ml).

10)   What is vital capacity?

-    The vital capacity is the total volume of air needed for vital exchanges.

Chapter 9

1) Is the vital capacity of a person with COPD increased or decreased?

- The vital capacity of a person with COPD is decreased.

2) What is atelectasis?

- Atelectasis is the collapse of the pulmonary alveoli.

3) Is atelectasis reversible?

- Yes, atelectasis is reversible.

4) Can the lungs be empty?

- No, the lungs are never empty. There is always the residual volume in the lungs.

5) What is polycythemia?

-      Polycythemia is an abnormality of the increase of erythrocytes.

6)   What is the function of erythrocytes?

-      Erythrocytes, also called red blood cells, their function is to carry oxygen.

7)   Is the level of erythrocyte higher or lower in a person with COPD?

-      The level of erythrocyte is higher in a person with COPD because there is an increase in erythrocyte production to fill the oxygen deficiency.

8)   What is the treatment of a COPD of viral origin?

-      The treatment of a COPD of viral origin is a bronchodilator treatment.

9)   What is the treatment of COPD of bacterial origin?

-       The treatment of COPD of bacterial origin is an antibiotic treatment.

10)   Do all exacerbations of COPD require antibiotic treatment?

-       No, not all exacerbations of COPD require antibiotic treatment.

Chapter 10

1) Why is it that not all exacerbations of COPD require antibiotic treatment?

- Not all exacerbations of COPD require antibiotic treatment as they are often limited local infections.

2) Can COPD be a genetic anomaly?

- Yes, COPD can be a genetic anomaly.

3) What is the cause of the genetic abnormality in COPD?

- The cause of the genetic abnormality in COPD is a deficit of alpha 1-antitrypsin.

4) What kind of diet is very important for people with COPD?

-      The kind of diet that is very important for people with COPD is a protein diet in order to develop muscles.

5)   Why should people with COPD be well hydrated?

-      People with COPD need to be well hydrated in order to make the mucus thinner.

6)   What are the side effects of corticosteroids?

-      The side effects of corticosteroids are hyperglycemia, osteoporosis, risk of infection, etc.

7)   What is osteoporosis?

-      Osteoporosis is the loss of bone density.

8)   Why are people taking corticosteroids at risk for infections?

-      People taking corticosteroids are at risk for infections because corticosteroids suppress the immune system.

9)   What is anticholinergic?

-      Anticholinergic is a substance that blocks the neurotransmitter acetylcholine in the central and peripheral nervous system.

10)   What are the functions of acetylcholine?

-      Acetylcholine is a neurotransmitter that causes contraction of skeletal muscles. It plays a role in sleep cycles and also plays a role in the endocrine system.

Conclusion

Thank you again for purchasing this book. I hope it has helped you in your journey to understanding COPD and how it affects the people around you who suffer from it.

Please, if you enjoyed this book, I would like you to leave a review. It'd be appreciated.

Thank you.

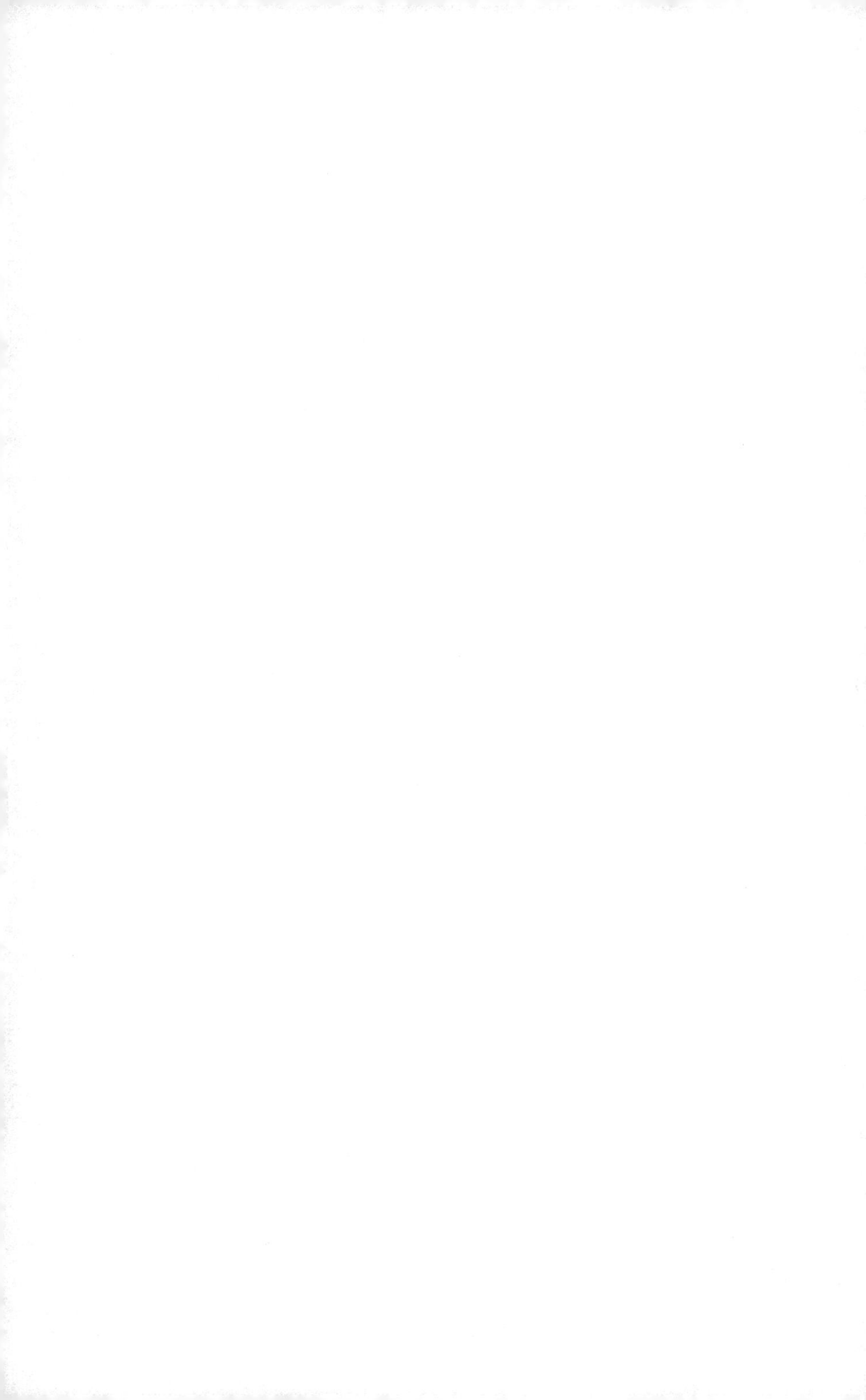